BUMP TRUTHS AND THE PREGNANT PAUSE: MYTHS, FACTS AND WHAT YOU REALLY NEED TO KNOW

WHY ONLY SHE ? WHY NOT HE ?

AUTHOR RIDDHIMA MAYANKA GAUR

To all the mothers — past, present, and future —
whose love begins before the first heartbeat is heard.

And to the babies, the silent teachers of strength, hope, and patience,
who remind us that life begins with belief, but flourishes with truth.

Contents

Foreword

Pregnancy has always been viewed through a lens of mystery and reverence — and rightfully so. It is a transformative phase in a woman's life, filled with joy, curiosity, and often, confusion. For centuries, societies across the world have passed down advice layered with tradition, emotion, and caution. Some of this wisdom has stood the test of time, while some has drifted into the realm of myth and misconception.

This book arrives as a gentle yet firm voice of clarity. It seeks to separate superstition from science and empower women with factual, reassuring, and compassionate guidance. Whether you are a first-time mom, a second-time learner, or a curious loved one — these pages aim to support, educate, and comfort you.

We live in an era where information is abundant, but truth is precious. This book helps you hold on to the truth — with calm confidence and a warm heart.

Preface

As the author of this book, I embarked on this journey with one simple goal: to create a trusted companion for every woman stepping into the life-changing journey of motherhood.

During my research and conversations with mothers, medical experts, and traditional caregivers, I realized how misinformation often travels faster than truth, especially during pregnancy. Harmless-sounding myths can cause unnecessary fear or guilt. That's when I felt a strong need to offer something meaningful — something honest.

This book is not a rulebook. It's a collection of myths gently unpacked, explained with facts, and balanced with cultural respect. It celebrates motherhood by encouraging awareness and understanding — without fear, shame, or judgment.

I hope this book becomes a gentle hand on your shoulder, a soft voice in moments of doubt, and a smile when you realize — you are doing just fine.

Acknowledgements

This book would not have been possible without the kindness, expertise, and inspiration of many beautiful souls:

To the doctors, nurses, and midwives who patiently answered my questions and corrected my assumptions.

To the mothers who generously shared their personal stories and let me peek into their world of hope, hesitation, and humor.

To my editorial team and friends who read and reread drafts with thoughtful eyes and hearts.

To my family, for their love, understanding, and encouragement during the many late nights this book was written.

Most importantly, I thank every reader — for believing that truth matters, especially when a new life depends on it.

Prologue

There is a quiet magic that surrounds pregnancy — a mix of wonder, expectation, and countless questions. With every new flutter, every shifting symptom, a mother starts building not just a baby, but a future. And in that beautiful, delicate process, she often finds herself surrounded by a flood of advice — not all of it helpful.

Whispers of "Don't do this," or "This means that," echo from every corner — friends, relatives, social media, even strangers. It becomes difficult to know what to believe. This book exists to answer that call for clarity.

In these pages, you'll walk through the most common myths told to pregnant women — and meet the science and truth that gently dismantle them. But more than just facts, you'll find reassurance, respect for culture, and a nurturing tone that holds your hand like a wise friend.

Pregnancy is not a puzzle to be solved. It's a path to be walked with care, knowledge, and trust in your inner strength. And this book — humbly — wishes to walk that path with you.

CHAPTER ONE

Quantity Of Food To Eat

? Myth 1: Pregnant women should eat for two.

? Fact:

This is a widely misunderstood belief. While it's true that pregnant women need more nutrients, it doesn't mean doubling calorie intake. In fact, during the first trimester, most women don't need any extra calories. By the second trimester, only about 300–350 extra calories are needed per day, and around 450 extra in the third. What's important is quality over quantity — eating foods rich in vitamins, minerals, fiber, protein, and healthy fats rather than simply increasing portion sizes.

CHAPTER TWO

Exercise During Pregnancy

⚥? **Myth 2: Exercise is dangerous during pregnancy.**
   ? Fact:
Unless a healthcare provider has advised against it due to specific conditions (like placenta previa or preterm labor risks), regular moderate exercise is beneficial. Activities like walking, swimming, prenatal yoga, and stretching help with circulation, muscle tone, mood, and even labor preparation. Exercise can also prevent gestational diabetes and reduce back pain. Always stay hydrated, avoid overheating, and listen to your body.

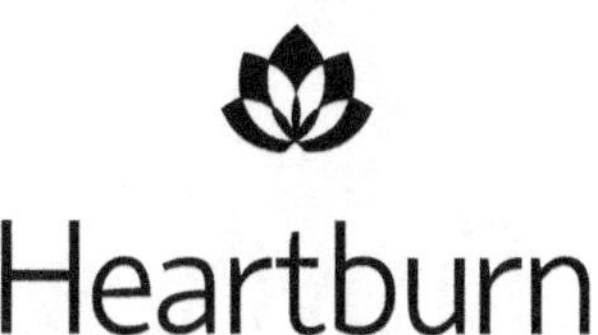

Heartburn

? Myth 3: Heartburn means your baby will have a lot of hair.

? Fact:

This amusing myth has been around for ages. Heartburn during pregnancy is typically due to hormonal changes (mainly increased progesterone) that relax the valve between the stomach and esophagus, causing acid reflux. As the uterus grows, it also puts pressure on the stomach, worsening the condition. Some studies have shown a slight correlation between maternal hormone levels and fetal hair growth, but it's far from definitive. So, don't take heartburn as a reliable hair predictor.

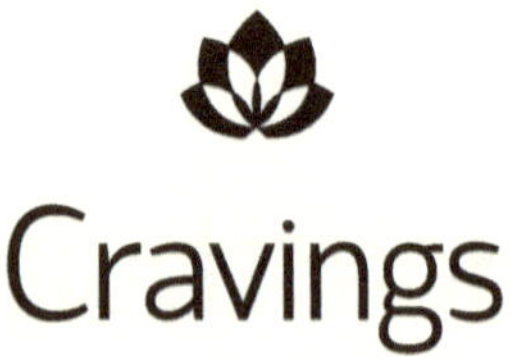

CHAPTER FOUR

Cravings

? Myth 4: Craving salty or sweet foods predicts the baby's gender.
   ? Fact:
Many believe that craving sweets means you're having a girl, while salty or savory cravings mean a boy. In reality, pregnancy cravings stem from hormonal fluctuations, nutritional needs, or emotional factors, not the baby's sex. The only reliable methods for gender determination include ultrasound, genetic testing, or birth.

CHAPTER FIVE

Caffeine Intake

? Myth 5: You can't have any caffeine during pregnancy.
   ? Fact:
Complete caffeine avoidance isn't necessary unless advised otherwise. However, excessive caffeine can increase the risk of miscarriage or low birth weight. Up to 200 mg of caffeine per day (about one 12-ounce cup of coffee) is generally considered safe. Be cautious of caffeine from other sources like tea, chocolate, energy drinks, and soft drinks.

CHAPTER SIX

Relaxing and Resting

?? Myth 6: Pregnant women should rest all the time.
  ? Fact:
Rest is important, especially when fatigued, but too much inactivity can cause issues like poor circulation, swelling, and blood clots. Moderate movement — such as daily walks, light housework, or stretching — keeps muscles active and improves mood and sleep. Always consult your doctor about activity levels, especially if complications arise.

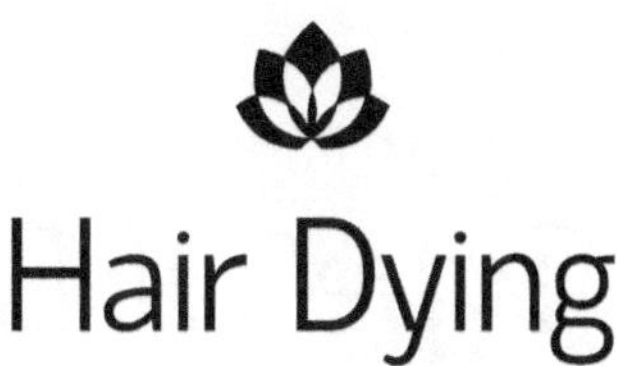

CHAPTER SEVEN

Hair Dying

? Myth 7: You shouldn't dye your hair when pregnant.
   ? Fact:
Most studies indicate that modern hair dyes contain low levels of chemicals that are unlikely to harm a developing fetus, especially when used occasionally. To be extra cautious, many women wait until after the first trimester. Use ammonia-free or natural dyes, and always apply in a well-ventilated space.

CHAPTER EIGHT

What Type Of Bath Is Good During Pregnancy

? Myth 8: Hot baths or saunas are safe in pregnancy.

? Fact:

Soaking in very hot water (above 100°F or 38°C), especially in early pregnancy, can increase the risk of neural tube defects and overheating. Saunas and hot tubs are generally discouraged. A warm bath is safe and relaxing as long as the temperature is comfortable and not too hot.

CHAPTER NINE

Visiting Dentist Doctor Is Safe or Not ?

? Myth 9: Visiting the dentist during pregnancy is unsafe.

? Fact:

Dental visits are not only safe but strongly recommended during pregnancy. Hormonal changes can cause swollen gums (pregnancy gingivitis) and increase the risk of infections. Inform your dentist about the pregnancy, and avoid unnecessary X-rays or elective procedures during the first trimester. Urgent dental care is essential for both mother and baby's health.

CHAPTER TEN

Is Traveling Safe or Not

? Myth 10: Traveling during pregnancy is dangerous.

? Fact:

Traveling is usually safe for most pregnant women up to about 36 weeks, unless the doctor advises against it. The second trimester (weeks 14–28) is often the most comfortable time to travel. Long trips should include frequent breaks to walk and stretch, stay hydrated, and wear seatbelts properly (below the belly). Air travel is also safe in most cases but check with your doctor and airline policies.

CHAPTER ELEVEN

Can Eclipses Harm

? **Myth 11: Eclipses can harm the baby.**

   ? **Fact:**

This is a cultural superstition found in many regions. Some believe that being outside during an eclipse may cause birth defects. Scientifically, there's no evidence supporting this. Eclipses are natural astronomical events with no impact on pregnancy or fetal development. Still, many women follow these customs out of respect for traditions or family beliefs.

CHAPTER TWELVE

Medications

? Myth 12: All medications are harmful during pregnancy.
  ? Fact:
While certain medications are unsafe and can harm fetal development, many others are safe and necessary. Never self-medicate or stop a prescribed drug without consulting a healthcare provider. For conditions like asthma, thyroid disorders, or infections, appropriate medication is crucial for the well-being of both mother and child.

CHAPTER THIRTEEN

Impact Of Stress During Pregnancy

⚥? Myth 13: Stress has no impact on the baby.

? Fact:

Chronic or intense stress can affect hormone levels in the body, potentially influencing the baby's brain development, birth weight, or triggering premature labor. Occasional stress is normal, but managing it through relaxation techniques, talking to loved ones, or seeking professional support can help maintain emotional and physical health.

CHAPTER FOURTEEN

Paint

? Myth 14: Pregnant women shouldn't be around paint.

? Fact:

Some types of paint contain harmful fumes like lead or solvents, which are risky if inhaled for long periods. However, using modern low-VOC, water-based paints in well-ventilated areas is generally safe. Wearing gloves and avoiding enclosed spaces further reduces any potential risks.

CHAPTER FIFTEEN

When Labor Pain Starts

? Myth 15: Old wives' tales can predict when labor will start.
  ? Fact:
Stories like labor beginning during a full moon, from eating spicy food, or when the mother starts cleaning obsessively are anecdotal and not scientifically supported. True signs of labor include regular contractions, water breaking, and cervical dilation. Always contact your healthcare provider when you suspect labor, rather than relying on folklore.

A Closing Note

? From Belief to Truth: A Final Word

Pregnancy is a sacred and emotional journey that transforms a woman not just physically, but emotionally and spiritually. Along this path, countless pieces of advice, cultural practices, and beliefs surround the expectant mother — some rooted in science, while others stem from tradition and hearsay.

In this guide, we aimed to shine a light on the common myths that are often accepted without question and may even pose risks to both the mother and child. More importantly, we presented facts based on medical expertise and scientific evidence, empowering every expectant mother to make informed and confident decisions.

? A Gentle Reminder: Every Pregnancy is Unique

No two pregnancies are the same. What works for one person might not be suitable for another. Therefore, it is vital to prioritize the advice of healthcare professionals over societal suggestions, online tips, or age-old customs.

? Purpose of This Guide

To provide clear, accurate, and reliable information

To help pregnant women rise above misconceptions and fear

To support the journey of becoming a strong, informed, and confident mother

♥? With You in This Beautiful Journey

Pregnancy is not just about growing a new life — it's also about growing as a person. Each day, each emotion, and each kick brings a new story. We hope this content brings clarity, reduces anxiety, and enriches your journey into motherhood

? Reach Out and Share

If you have questions, feedback, or personal experiences to share, we would love to hear from you. Every mother's voice matters — and it deserves to be heard.

? Wishing You and Your Little One All the Best!

"Step into motherhood with wisdom — because an informed mother is the best mother."